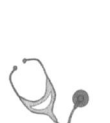

This is an IndieMosh book

brought to you by MoshPit Publishing
an imprint of Mosher's Business Support Pty Ltd

PO Box 4363
Penrith NSW 2750

indiemosh.com.au

Copyright © Russell Gruen 2022

The moral right of the author has been asserted in accordance with the Copyright Amendment (Moral Rights) Act 2000.

All rights reserved. Except as permitted under the Australian Copyright Act 1968 (for example, fair dealing for the purposes of study, research, criticism or review) no part of this publication may be reproduced, stored in a retrieval system, or transmitted in any form or by any means, electronic, mechanical, photocopying, recording or otherwise, without the written permission of the publisher.

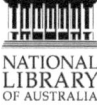 A catalogue record for this work is available from the National Library of Australia

https://www.nla.gov.au/collections

Title:	The Wise Doctor
Author:	Gruen, Russell (1968–)
ISBNs:	9781922812094 (paperback) 9781922812100 (ebook – epub) 9781922812117 (ebook – Kindle)
Subjects:	MEDICAL / Education & Training EDUCATION / Philosophy, Theory & Social Aspects

This book is not intended as a substitute for the career advice of recognised institutions and official mentors/trainers. And while every care has been taken with the publication of this book, the author and publisher accept no liability to any party for any loss, damage or disruption caused by errors or omissions, whether such errors or omissions result from negligence, accident or any other cause.

Illustrated by Holly Jones

Cover design and layout by Sarah Davies at www.instagram.com/lemon.design.studios

The Wise Doctor

by Russell Gruen

Illustrated by Holly Jones

For those who came before me,
who showed what it is to be a wise doctor.

For those who follow,
to find joy in becoming so.

And for those alongside,
with whom I share the journey.

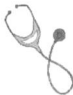

An earlier version of the ideas in this book
was published in the *British Journal of Surgery*
with Michael Hollands and David Watters,
both former presidents of
the Royal Australasian College of Surgeons
and who both embody wisdom in its fullest expression.

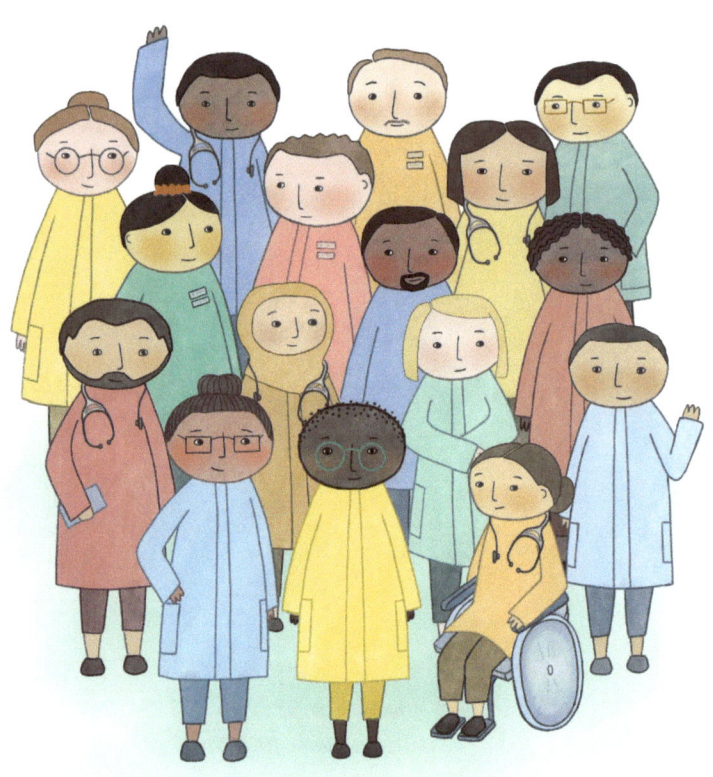

The best doctors are recognisable by more than technical excellence and superior knowledge, essential as these attributes are. Although often senior, it is more than age and experience that distinguishes them. They are the colleagues from whom others seek advice because they make good decisions. They willingly provide guidance and support. Their actions match their opinions, and their outcomes justify their practice. They appreciate the context and drivers of doubt confronting any choice, and their advice is grounded in common sense. They provide mentorship for peers and juniors, and indeed are sought out to do so. We might say such doctors are wise, and it is their wisdom that we admire.

This small book addresses wisdom in medicine, in the hope that doctors will aspire to it, educators will champion it, clinics will foster it, and people everywhere will be better for it.

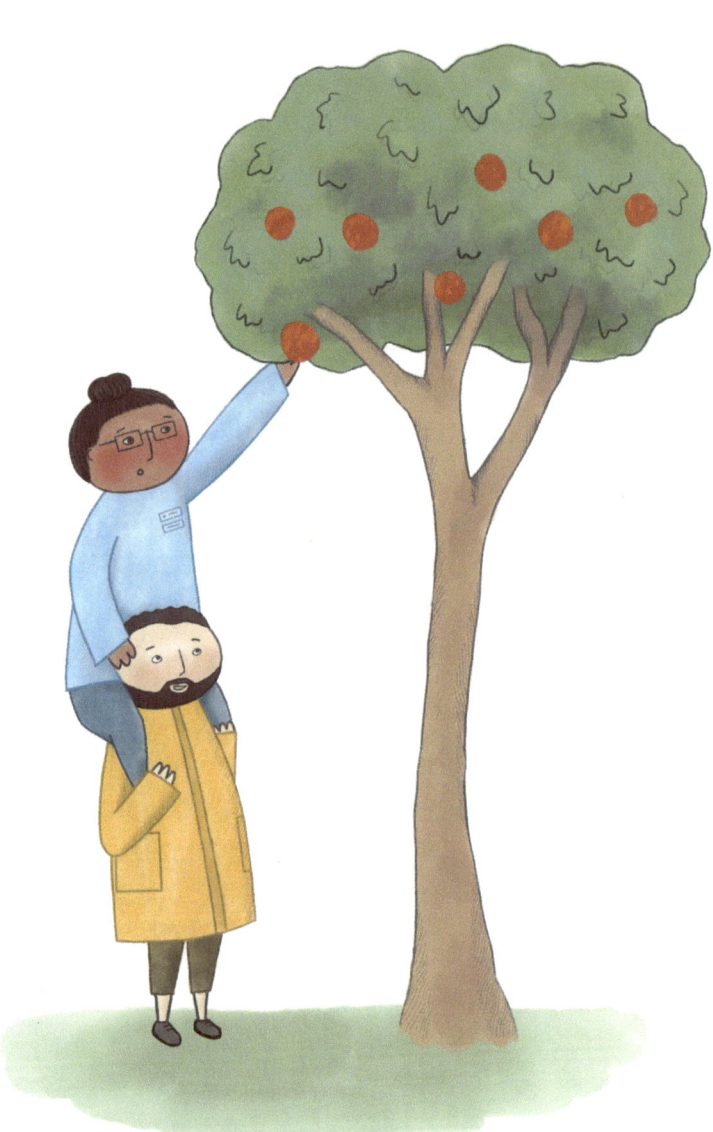

What is wisdom?

Wisdom is a complex human trait that transcends generation and culture. It embodies elements of rational decision-making, general knowledge of life, empathy, compassion and altruism, comprehension of divergent values, emotional stability, insight or self-reflection, and the ability to proceed and progress in the face of uncertainty.

For centuries people have sought to understand wisdom, and how to be wise. Aristotle offered a practical view. Being wise, he argued, requires the ability to see, on each occasion, which course of action is best supported by reason. And by doing so, a wise person 'lives well'.

To Aristotle this ability has intellectual and moral underpinnings, grows with experience and time, is determined by choice and is acquired by habit.

Just as one who makes good decisions in life 'lives well', we can say that a doctor who consistently chooses the best course of action 'practises well'. What is it, then, that makes a doctor wise?

Being wise requires the ability to see which course of action is best supported by reason.

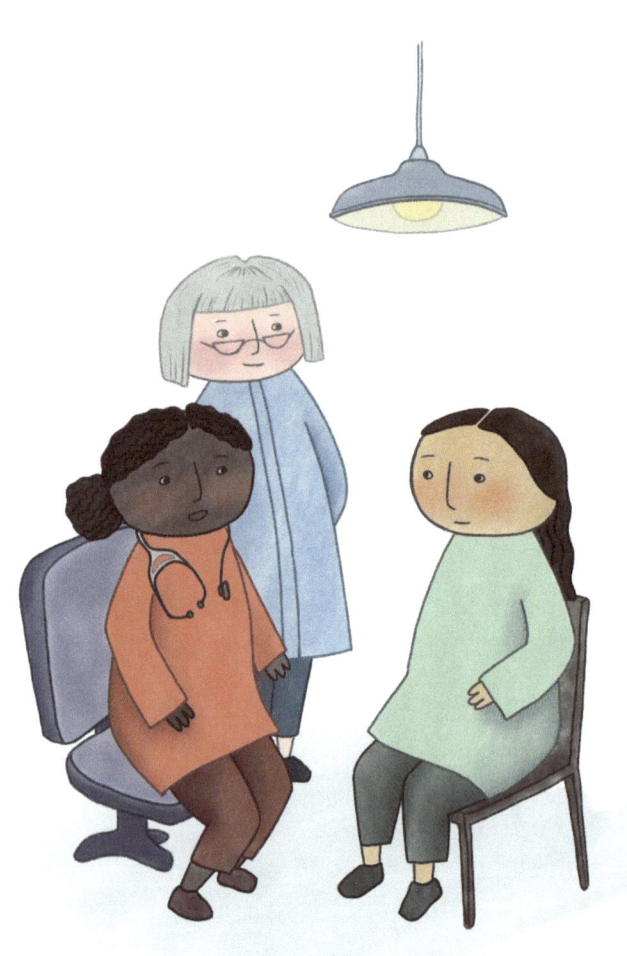

Competence and professionalism

Competence and professionalism are prerequisites for wise practice.

Competence encompasses the knowledge, skills and attitudes that are needed to be a doctor. Most medical training programs have competency-based frameworks for technical and non-technical skills, decision-making, communication, collaboration and teamwork, management and leadership. Much has been done to define, teach and assess such competencies.

Medical students won't graduate until they can treat patients with heart failure, for example, and surgical trainees won't qualify without being able to safely remove an infected gallbladder, or repair a broken bone. Each must understand the relevant science, be able to communicate effectively with people, and demonstrate the ability to work with other members of the healthcare team.

Medical professionalism refers to the moral, cognitive and collegial aspects of being a doctor. Professionalism includes such things as putting patients' interests first, even if it means attending at inconvenient times, or recommending a course of action that doesn't attract a doctor's fee.

It includes honesty, even when it is uncomfortable, such as when mistakes are made or treatment doesn't go as planned. It includes respecting patients' autonomy, even when they make choices we wouldn't make ourselves, and their right to confidentiality, even if they aren't within earshot to hear us talking about them. At its heart lies integrity: doing the right thing, without cutting corners, even when we're tired and when nobody is watching.

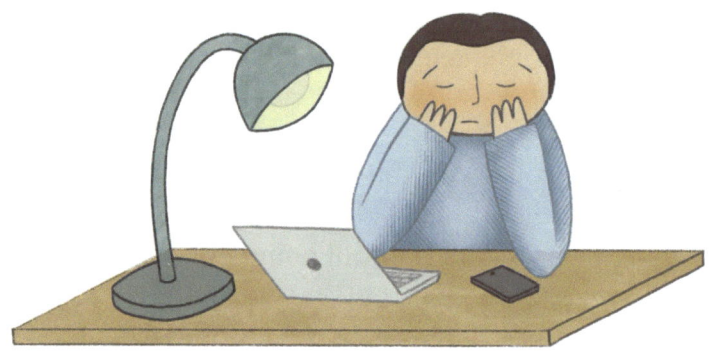

Beyond how we relate to patients, professionalism also refers to how we work respectfully with colleagues, especially when their opinions differ from our own, and how we contribute our expertise in broader public discourse about health-related issues.

All of this is underpinned by what has been referred to as a 'social contract' that doctors and other professionals have with the society we serve, in which the trust people bestow, the regard in which professionals are held and the privileges we enjoy are conditional on our professional behaviour.

Neither incompetence nor unprofessional behaviour is acceptable, so it follows that competence and professionalism are the minimum expected by patients, peers, regulators and the public.

But medical wisdom is something more.

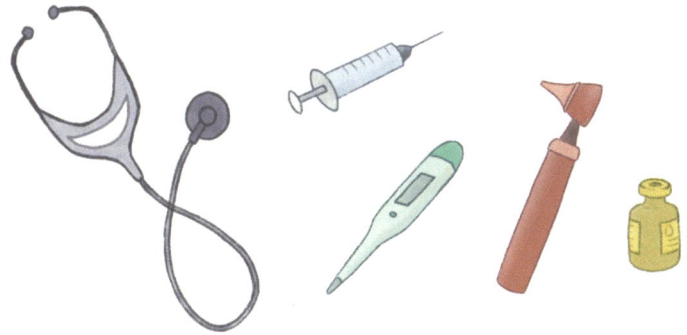

The difference seems to lie in four additional attributes that, together, enable the wise doctor to consistently choose the best course of action.

These attributes are superior judgement, rich understanding, few unjustified beliefs and a strong moral compass.

Competence and professionalism are minimum expectations. Medical wisdom is something more.

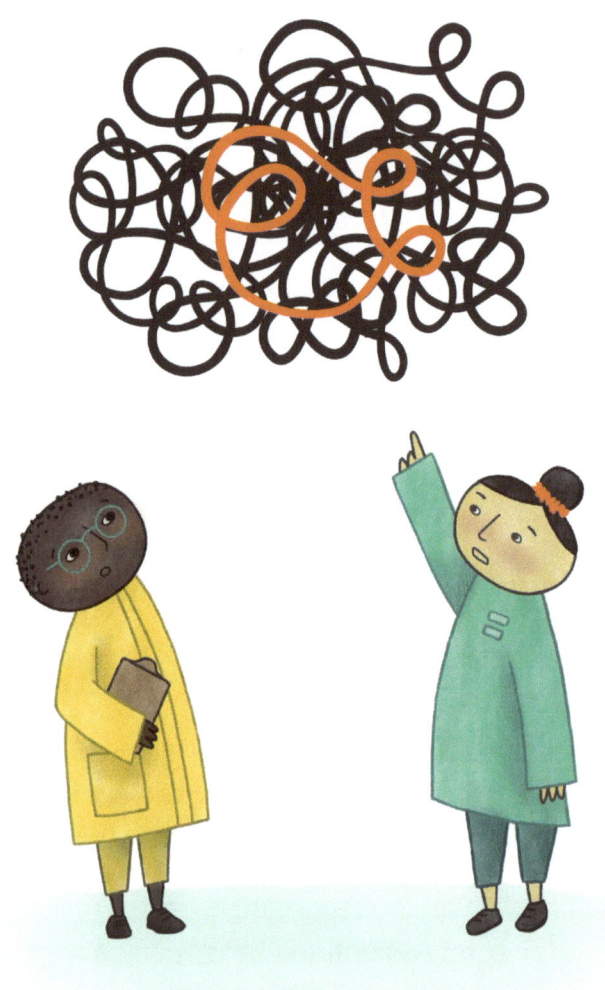

Superior judgement

At the core of most definitions of wisdom is the ability to judge truly what is right or fitting in any situation, and to perceive and adopt the best means for accomplishing an end. Even when we're confronted with unfamiliar challenges, risks and probabilities must be considered, and behaviours contextualised.

So in our own moments of indecision we're likely to wonder, 'What would a wise doctor do in this situation?'

Doctors who consistently make good decisions necessarily have excellent clinical skills and situational awareness. They consider all the options, and they thrive on detail and nuance.

The best diagnostic and treatment plans take into account specific characteristics of the illness and other concerns that patients may have, the available family and carer support, and how successful patients are likely to be with treatment requirements. The best plans also take into account characteristics of the treating team and how well they match each patient's needs.

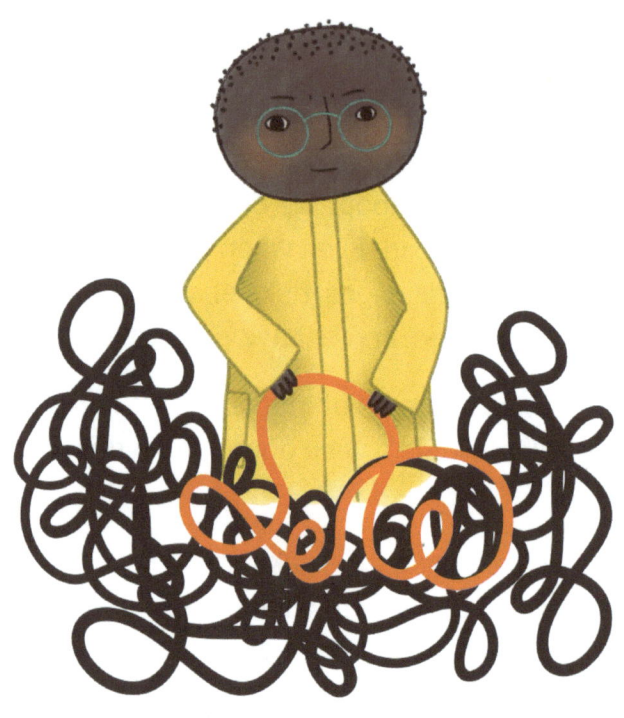

For example, there are many medication options for treating high blood pressure in patients with multiple medical problems. There is more than one combination of surgery and radiotherapy from which patients with breast cancer who live far from the treating hospital can choose. There are several approaches, ranging from exercise to surgery, for helping elderly patients live with arthritis, pain and limited mobility. The wise doctor helps to choose the best option each time.

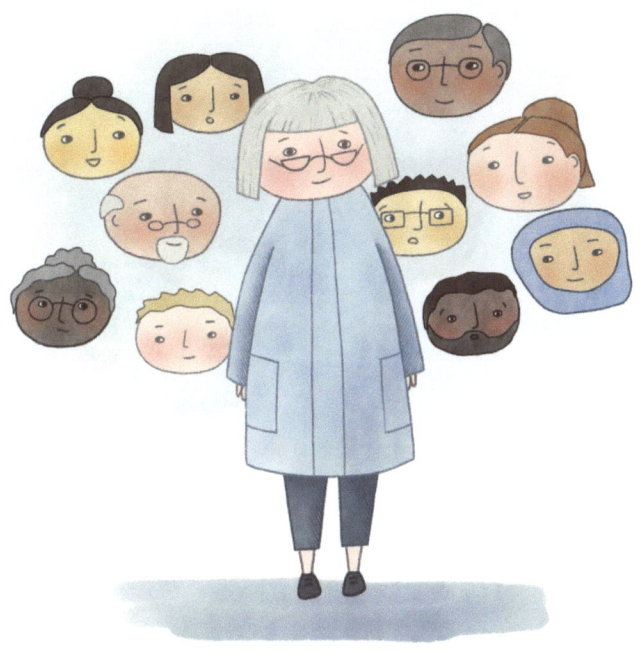

Seamless situational assessment and action planning may seem like 'intuition,' a characteristic of experts who have navigated intricate and perplexing situations many times before. In doing so, they've developed cognitive scripts: organised compilations of relevant knowledge gained through learning and experience, often accessed subconsciously. Their intuition is, rather, the rapid and confident retrieval of appropriate information.

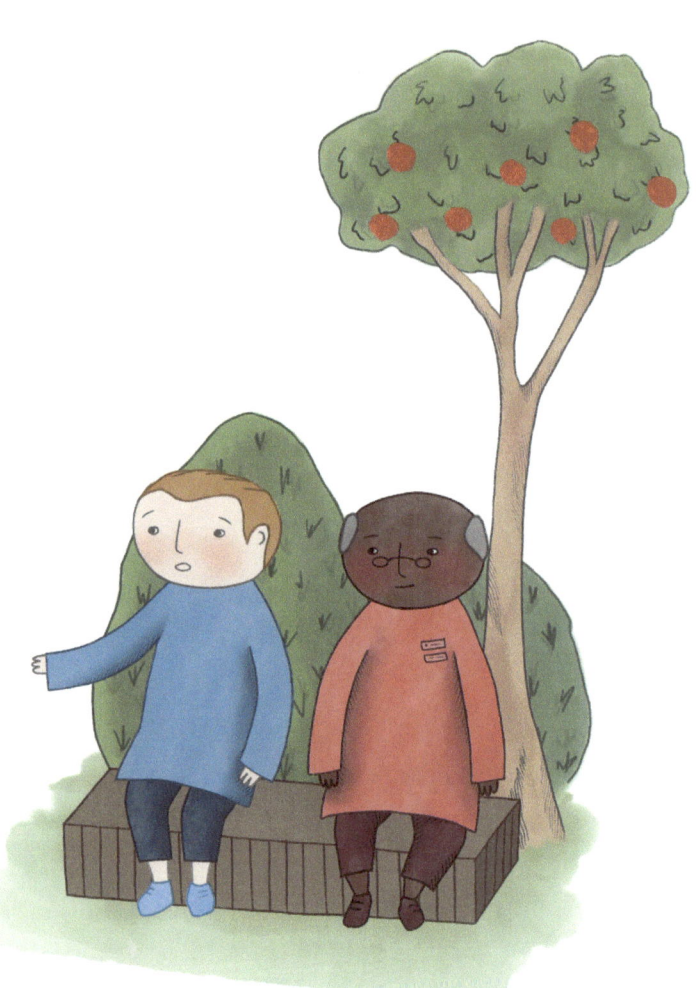

Rich understanding

To Aristotle, 'living well' requires a rich understanding of the nature of things and how they fit together as a whole. Wise doctors make good decisions in part because they understand 'the ways in which the world works', including the nature of health and disease, the role of prevention and treatment, the contributions made by different types of health professionals and informal carers, the capabilities of local services, and the complexities of healthcare delivery systems.

A wise doctor understands what healthcare means for patients ... what they must go through, including pain and other side effects, emotional upheaval, inconvenience, disruption and loss of independence. Undergoing surgery, for example, is an ordeal patients are usually willing to endure only because they perceive the need for rescue from something worse.

Rich understanding of peoples' health and wellbeing, healthcare, and patients' experiences comes from the social sciences and human psychology as well as the biomedical sciences. And it may lead some doctors to complement their healing and caregiving roles with prevention, advocacy and leadership activities.

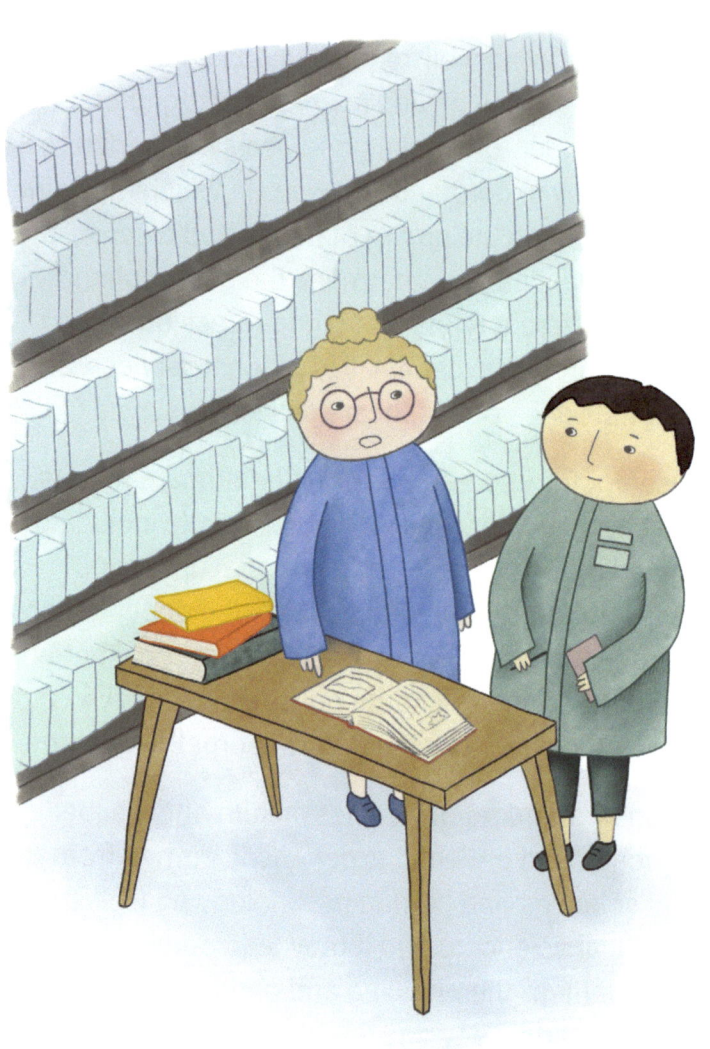

Few unjustified beliefs

Another way of thinking about being wise is that it's the opposite of being foolish. People can be foolish when they believe or state things that aren't true, or do things that aren't warranted. In contrast, wise people can justify their beliefs through fact, experience or reason.

It follows that unwise doctors have unjustified beliefs, stemming from a poor knowledge base and misguided trust in unfounded approaches. They may also be unaware how well their outcomes compare to others', or ambivalent towards doing what is best.

On the other hand, wise doctors have good knowledge of what works and what doesn't, and can justify their reasoning. They have few unjustified beliefs.

Furthermore, they are aware that everyone's expertise has limits. Wise doctors know when they step outside the boundaries of personal competence, and when it's best to consult a colleague.

Wise doctors have good knowledge of what works, and can justify their reasoning.

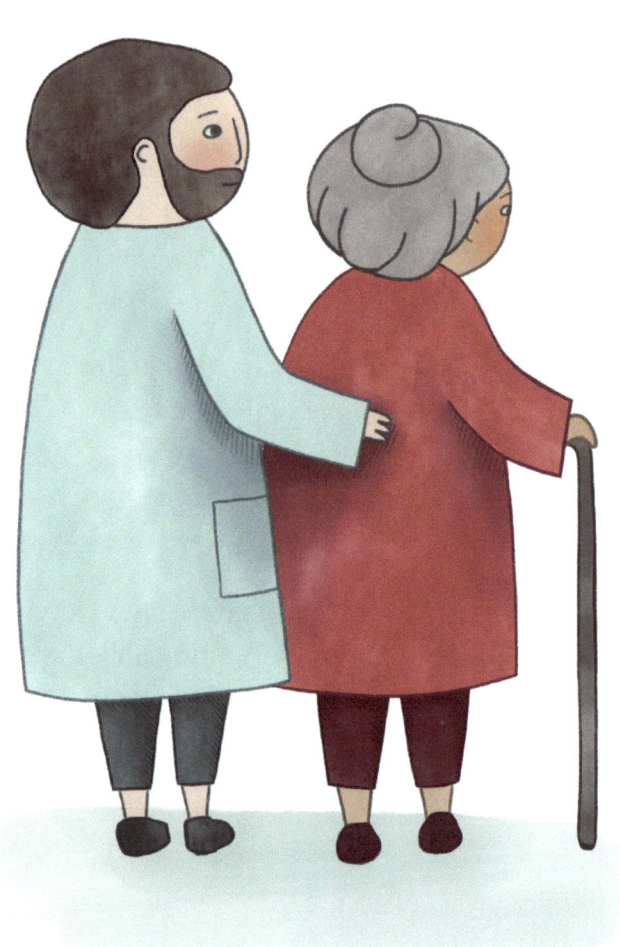

A strong moral compass

Along with its practical application, Aristotle regarded wisdom as the ultimate expression of virtue, or moral excellence. Virtue originates in our innermost thoughts and desires. It determines what we value, and the beliefs, ideas and opinions that come to represent a personal ethic.

Moral excellence and integrity, not just rigid beliefs, guide wise doctors toward right and good actions. When we're making difficult and complex decisions, our patients' interests usually guide us to moral true north.

Wisdom requires not just having good values and ethics, but also living and modelling those values, perhaps better described as 'walking the talk'.

Living our values may be especially challenging when we're busy and tired. Wise doctors manage themselves as well as they do their patients.

When faced with difficult decisions, it is our patients' interests that mark true north.

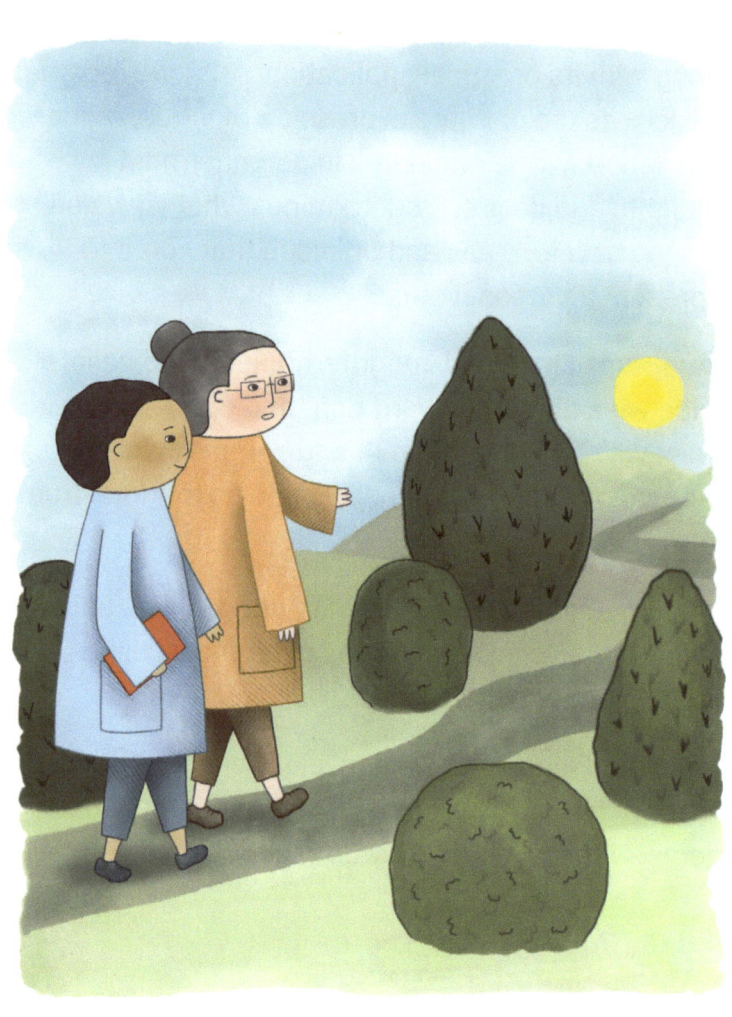

Becoming wise

Completion of training signifies competence for clinical practice and, throughout our careers, doctors are expected to continue to learn and develop expertise.

Yet wisdom is not just layers of experience on a core of taught competencies. Nor is it attained solely by learning and following general rules.

Rather, wisdom is an emergent property of highly integrated brain functioning, developed through upbringing and habit.

Superior judgement requires deliberative, emotional and social skills refined by solving problems many times over. We can accelerate this learning through combinations of scenario-based training, simulation and reflective practice.

Rich understanding comes from thinking deeply, from curiosity and questioning. Our classrooms and workplaces should be places of enquiry and critique, where staff and students share ideas and challenge assumptions.

Doctors who have **few unjustified beliefs** habitually read, analyse, reflect and welcome feedback. They know the latest evidence in their field, and what it means for the care they offer patients, and they hold themselves to account by auditing their performance, identifying gaps and opportunities for improvement.

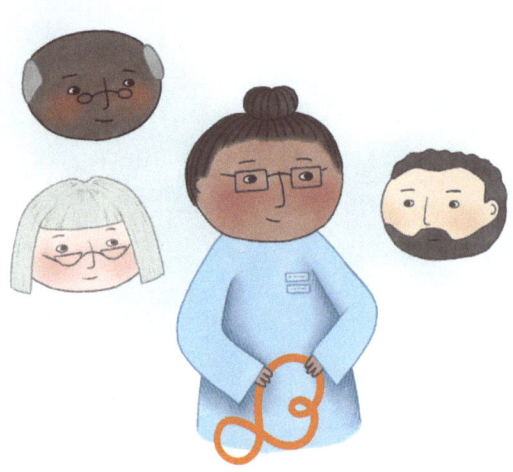

Values that underpin a **strong moral compass** are fostered through explicit commitment to patients' welfare. Aligned organisational values, consistent behaviour expectations and good role models can illuminate the path.

Wisdom can't be learnt, nor does it come just with experience. It develops with time, and depends on choices and habits.

Best-in-class doctors are more than competent and professional. They make good decisions because they have attained a rich understanding of the nature of things. They're motivated by what is true and right. And they have heightened acumen through critical reflection and self-improvement.

This combination of qualities, embodying professional attributes and individual ethos, personifies the wise doctor.

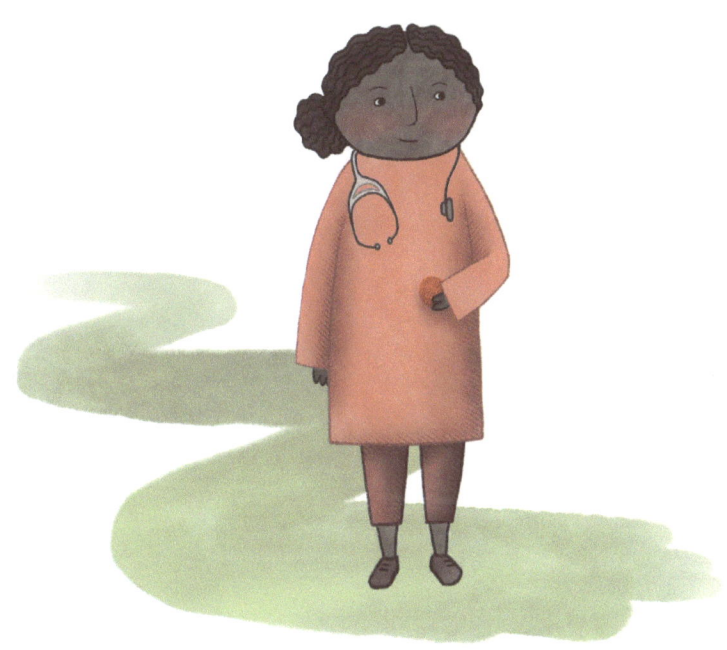

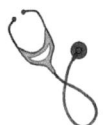

Suggested further reading

Practical wisdom

Aristotle. Nicomachean ethics. In: The basic works of Aristotle, McKeon R (ed.) Random House: New York, 1941;935–1112.

Meeks TW, Jeste DV. Neurobiology of wisdom: a literature overview. Arch Gen Psychiatry 2009;66:355–365.

Competence and professionalism

Royal College of Physicians and Surgeons of Canada. The CanMEDS Physician Competency Framework. https://www.royalcollege.ca/rcsite/canmeds/about-canmeds-e

Medical Professionalism Project. Medical professionalism in the new millennium: a physicians' charter. Lancet 2002;359(9305):520–522.

American College of Surgeons Task Force on Professionalism. Professionalism in surgery. J Am Coll Surg 2003;197:605–608.

Superior judgement

Groopman JE. How doctors think. Houghton Mifflin: Boston, 2007.

Kaldjian LC. Teaching practical wisdom in medicine through clinical judgement, goals of care, and ethical reasoning. J Med Ethics 2010;36:558–562.

Abernathy C, Hamm RM. Surgical intuition: What it is and how to get it. Hanley & Belfus: Philadelphia, 1995.

Kneebone R. Expert. Viking: London, 2020.

Rich understanding

Boudreau JD, Cassell EJ. Medical wisdom. Perspect Biol Med 2021;64(2):251–270.

Little JM. Ethics in surgical practice. Br J Surg 2001;88:769–770.

Flin R, O'Connor P, Crichton M. Safety at the sharp end: a guide to non-technical skills. CRC Press: Boca Raton, FL, 2008.

Few unjustified beliefs

Sackett DL, Rosenberg WMC, Gray JAM, Haynes RB, Richardson WS. Evidence based medicine: What it is and what it isn't. BMJ 1996;312:71.

Kamtchum-Tatuene J, Zafack JG. Keeping up with the medical literature: Why, how, and when? Stroke 2021;52(11):e746–8.

NHS. Audit and service improvement, 2021. https://www.nice.org.uk/about/what-we-do/into- practice/audit-and-service-improvement

A strong moral compass

Pellegrino ED, Thomasma DC. The virtues in medical practice. Oxford University Press: New York, 1993.

Gruen RL, Pearson SE, Brennan TA. Physician-Citizens: public roles and professional obligations. JAMA 2004;291(1):94–8.

A previous version of these ideas

Gruen RL, Watters DAK, Hollands MJ. Surgical wisdom. Br J Surg 2012;99(1):3–5.

About the author

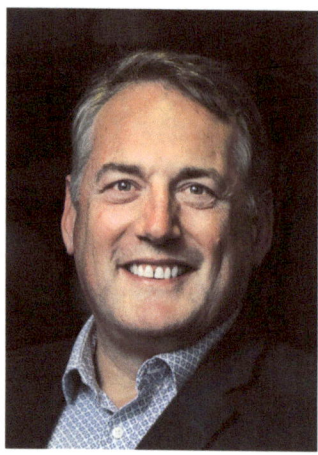

Professor Russell Gruen is the Dean of the College of Health and Medicine at the Australian National University. A surgeon who has worked in Australia, the US and Singapore, he embodies thirty years of insights from thousands of patients and their families. As a trauma specialist he performed life-saving emergency surgery, led multidisciplinary teams, and supported severely injured people to rebuild their lives.

Having also completed a doctoral degree on access to healthcare in Australian outback communities, and with further training in health policy, medical ethics and business management at Harvard, Russell brings a broad perspective to strengthening health systems, developing leaders, and advancing the profession of medicine.

Russell and his wife, a family doctor, have two sons.

About the illustrator

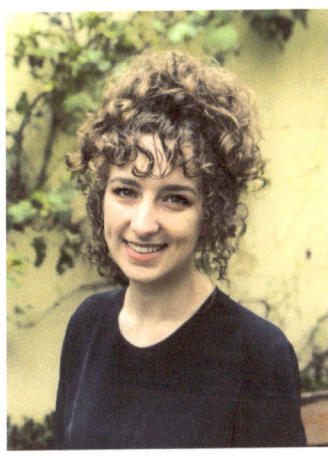

Holly Jones is a Canberra-based visual artist who uses texture, depth and colour to convey meaning, and structure and subtle connections to create narrative. Her chronic medical condition was the catalyst for her artistic practice over the last seven years, during which she developed a deep appreciation of the impact that wise doctoring can have on an individual's quality of life.

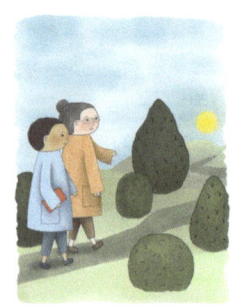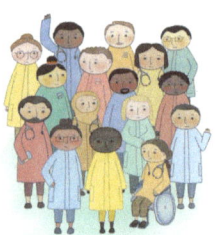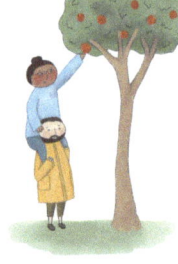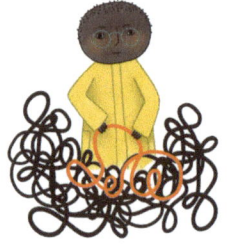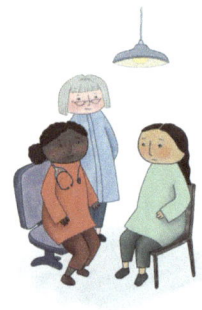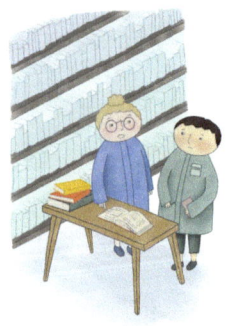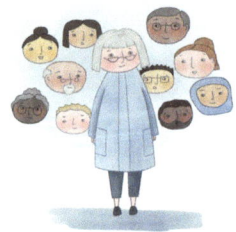

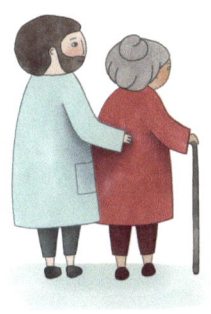
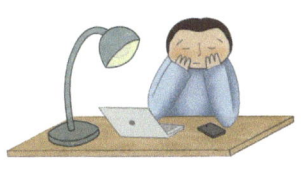
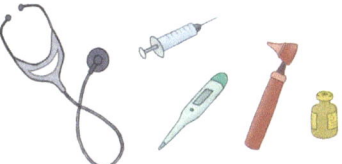
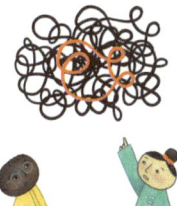
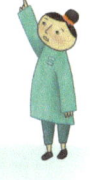
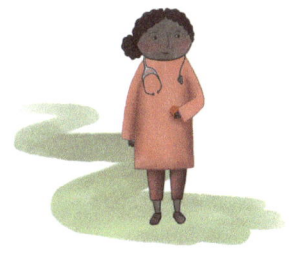
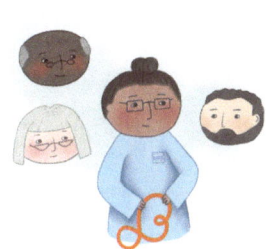
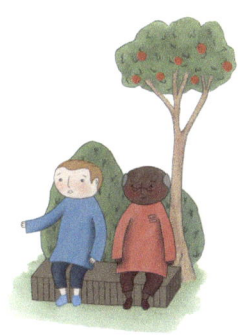

www.ingramcontent.com/pod-product-compliance
Lightning Source LLC
LaVergne TN
LVHW070438080526
838202LV00038B/2842